Pressing
RESET
—— for the ——
Triathlete

ᕯoriginal
strength

Original strength

Pressing RESET for the Triathlete

Published by OS Press - Fuquay-Varina, NC

Contributor: Jackie Miller USAT Level III Coach - FMS Level 2 Certified- Original Strength Certified PRO - ACE Personal Trainer - https://www.britfit.com/

ISBN: 979-8-9865860-9-0 (Paperback)

I wrote this booklet because I believe in this system.

It works.

My practice, both within my business application and racing career accomplishments, upholds that point.

I am grateful for the continuous learning opportunities provided by the OS community. I feel fortunate to have had the chance to meet and work alongside Tim Anderson, the innovator behind the Original Strength System, over twenty years ago.

Within every training plan I write or every training session I teach, the RESETs are a constant.

RESETs are inherent movements that come naturally to you. Utilizing these movements can enhance the systems you depend on, whether you are new to triathlons or a seasoned professional preparing to compete internationally.

I am sharing this information because, as a successful competitor, multi-sports events require a lot of movement.

So the question I have for you is: How *well* do you move?

The training for a multi-sport event regularly requires you to do two-a-day workouts – and that can be a lot to handle! Swimming, biking, running, and strength conditioning work are necessary to achieve the endurance, durability, and resilience a triathlon demands. Those demands are quite taxing on several of your body systems – the physical, the mental, and the neurological.

Your training stress can affect the quality of your movement patterns and overall health. The triathlete's consistent training load can be challenging on many levels. The muscular-skeletal frame and neurological systems are constantly under stress. On top of that, we add in the stresses of our daily life activities.

Soon enough, the way we move and even breathe can sometimes become less than optimal; this leaves our ability to find restorative recovery difficult to harness. We get burnt out, sick, or worse still – injured.

With that bright future ahead of you, there is hope! In this booklet are RESETs that, if you choose to follow, can help save you from the negative 'stuff.' They can help you refresh and restore the natural movements you were born with.

You were born with these RESETs. The term 'Pressing RESET' is just what you do when you use these RESETs, or movement patterns, to help you move the way you were designed to move through your world.

Used as a warm-up, cool-down, movement preparation, or an actual workout, when combined together in a way that adds load or duration, these RESETs can be your next step towards all the good things you are training for.

By Pressing RESET, you can restore your Original Strength. You can be more resilient, both physically and mentally. You can relearn skills to help you handle stressful situations and meet the demands of your sport. Through practice, these simple RESETs can free up restrictions in movement patterns. Because we are a sum of many moving parts, when you free up one restriction, movement patterns can change in a good way.

> **By Pressing RESET, you can restore your Original Strength. You can be more resilient, both physically and mentally.**

Swimming, biking, and running are all complex sequences of movement patterns. Though you may be moving a lot, you may not be moving *well a lot*. Your movement quality is based on, for the most part, your musculoskeletal frame. However, the messenger driving the movement needs to be healthy and clear, too.

Therefore, you must have a healthy Autonomic Nervous System (ANS).

RESETs can help restore and nourish your ANS.

Within this system are the Sympathetic (fight, tense up, and flight) State and the Parasympathetic (rest, relax and digest) State. For your optimal performance and health, you need to learn ways to regulate these.

With daily RESET practice, a healthier nervous system can lead to all kinds of great things - like better sleep for recovery and healing, a higher capacity towards adaptation to your training, and simply just feeling better.

*Medical Disclaimer: It is important to note that we are not here to diagnose or treat any medical or physical disorder. This is meant to be a guide to developing the skills to participate in a triathlon and should not supersede any medical advice from your doctor or other health professionals that you work with. Do not move into pain. Pain is an alarm system telling your body that something is or may be wrong and needs to be respected. Our bodies compensate and move very differently when we are in pain. As we move more and better, your body should improve, but **if you cannot perform the movements in this guide without pain, then seek a medical professional.***

How You Can Press RESET

You were born with a reset button; it's wired into each of us.

The RESETs are part of the natural developmental sequence of human movement developed through your earliest years as a baby, then as a growing toddler, and on. They are simple and easy to follow. Daily practice is ideal, even if you do five to ten minutes worth of RESETs daily!

You will find several examples of ways to combine RESETs and create simple routines later in this book, along with some workout routine ideas.

Let's start by understanding what you should include as you Press RESET.

Pressing
RESET

The Three Pillars of Human Movement

By engaging in The Three Pillars of Human Movement, you can be a better version of your triathlete self. These pillars nourish your nervous system, providing many health and movement benefits. To do this, you should always:

1. Breathe with your diaphragm.
2. Activate your vestibular system.
3. Engage in contralateral movement patterns (gait patterning movements, crossing midline).

Let's understand a little more about these Three Pillars.

1. Diaphragm Breathing

You were more than likely born a natural diaphragmatic breather. You breathed using 'belly' breaths. However, it seems as the stress of life increases, we forget how to do that.

The diaphragm is a dome-shaped muscle. Think of it as an umbrella shape that opens as we inhale and closes as we exhale.

Its position separates the torso into the sections of the chest and abdomen. It is connected to the spine, ribcage, muscles, and organs.

Our breath, whether fast and shallow or deep and full, can activate our nervous system in a favorable or not-so-favorable way.

The way you breathe plays a huge role in how you train and race – from bolstering your ability to cope mentally as you face a choppy open water swim to staying focused on your race day plan on a windy day.

Breathing deeply - out and in - also restores movement within the approximately one hundred joints of your twelve pairs of ribs. This ribcage mobility is extremely beneficial on many counts. The structure of your ribcage affects your neck, spine, shoulders, and more. That can help you feel more comfortable in many aspects of your sport. After all, lifting your head to see where you are during the swim can take its toll, as can simply looking ahead of you while in aero on the bike.

Nasal breathing is encouraged when Pressing RESET. This is done by closing the mouth and placing the tongue in its resting position, at the roof of the mouth. Just by diaphragm breathing, you can:

- Clear stale air and carbon dioxide out.
- Draw oxygen deeper into the Alveoli air sacs within the lungs.

- Deliver more oxygen to the working muscles.
- Free up joint movement in the upper torso.
- Improve your form and technique for all three sports.
- Remain calmer in the face of a stressful situation.

2. The Vestibular System

The Vestibular System (VS) is fully developed within the womb at around 21 days. The VS, situated within your brain, receives messages from throughout the body.

In vertebrates, it is a sensory system that creates the sense of balance and spatial orientation, known as proprioception, for the purpose of coordinating movement with balance. It interprets how you move through your world. It even helps keep your eyes on the horizon.

As a very young baby, you instinctively 'trained' yourself by lifting and turning your head to see things around you. As you moved more, your system grew. With your developing head movements, used to roll you over to your belly or to your back, you naturally nurtured this developing organ.

A healthy VS plays a vital role in your movement efficiency.

You test your VS daily with your training when you swim, bike, and run. You constantly challenge it to help you keep your balance no matter where your body and head are.

During your training and racing, there will be a point when you are simply too tired to focus hard on your form. The better you maintain optimal posture, the less energy is wasted. Or the quicker you can react to running on uneven ground, the less chance you have of twisting an ankle.

> **You will have a reflexive 'backup system' by engaging in daily RESETs that include engaging your VS.**

Your ability to achieve these and more requires self-awareness and a healthy Vestibular System.

You will have a reflexive 'backup system' by engaging in daily RESETs that include engaging your VS.

3. Engage in Contralateral Movement Patterns

When you were born, you were already wired to crawl. Crawling is your gait pattern. It should be contralateral, which means moving while using anatomical opposition. In other words, the opposite sides of the body work together to coordinate the right arm and left leg and the left arm and right leg.

As a baby, you instinctively start to move about your new world contralaterally by first rolling.

As your strength and curiosity grew, you went from rolling to rocking and, eventually, crawling.

Your crawling activated your brain, and vital skills such as hand-eye coordination were developed. Your little body grew stronger as you were able to spend more time moving around. After all, you were born to move!

Daily RESETs that have contralateral patterns reinforce your gait patterning in many ways. **"Firing the wiring,"** or this brain plasticity, is beneficial and goes a long way toward your training demands.

Regular practice of this movement pattern can improve your efficiency as a triathlete. Swimming, biking, and running all require a counterbalance of your moving limbs. This forces the core to respond in a good way reflexively.

Many of the RESETs are contralateral, so it's easy to do. After all, if a baby can do it, shouldn't you be able to do it?

Pressing RESET with The Five RESETs

So, how do we Press RESET?

Including the Three Pillars of human movement as we Press RESET is easy. We include diaphragmatic breathing, awareness of your head (and eye) movement, and adding in gait patterning movements.

As mentioned earlier, you were born to move. These five things are already somewhere deep in your brain's memory banks. You probably rolled, rocked, and crawled. These movements developed your strength, proprioception, balance, and coordination.

The Big Five RESETS

1. **Diaphragmatic Breathing**
2. **Head Control**
3. **Rolling**
4. **Rocking**
5. **Crawling and contralateral, midline crossing movements**

When used as part of your daily practice, the way in which you move and how you feel you move will be different, hopefully in a better way.

We will go through each RESET and later learn how you can put them all together. Going for a certain amount of time can be a good metric so you meet where you are daily. Routines of the following RESETs can be used as a warm-up to a workout. They can be programmed and even loaded for a strength session or practiced daily to help you move and feel better.

Pressing
RESET

Diaphragmatic Breathing

Why?

- The diaphragm is a spinal stabilizer when pressurized. This helps support and protect your spine.

- This loading also helps maintain a strong pelvic floor.

- A strong diaphragm allows for deeper inhale and exhale for better gaseous exchange.

- Correct breathing can help restore a healthy nervous system.

How?

Movement Position #1

FACE DOWN OR PRONE POSITION

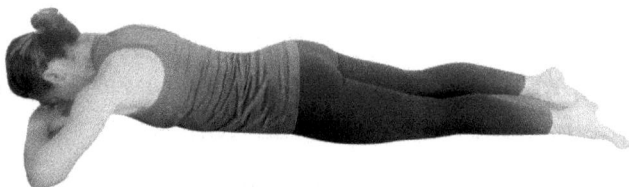

- Lie face down, resting your forehead on your hands.
- Lips closed, gently place your tongue on the roof of the mouth.
- Breathe out and in through your nose.
- Exhale, inhale, and repeat for 1-2 minutes.
- Notice your lower back area rise and fall.

Movement Position #2

SEATED QUADRUPED POSITION

The seated quadruped replicates your bike position.

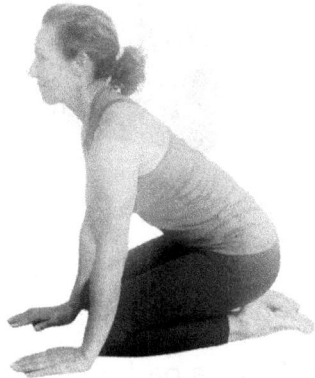

- Kneel on the floor with your hands beneath your shoulders and knees beneath your hips. Rock back and keep the hips back over that six-point position. Place a pad under the knees for comfort and either point the toes straight backward or curl the toes forward.

- Look towards the horizon.

- Lips closed, gently place your tongue on the roof of the mouth.

- Breathe out and in through your nose.

- Exhale, inhale, and repeat for 1-2 minutes.

- Gently allow the hips to open and sink lower; don't force them.

- Gently allow the ankles and feet to stretch.

- Notice the pressure downwards on your pelvic floor.

Movement Position #3

SIDE LYING 90-90 POSITION

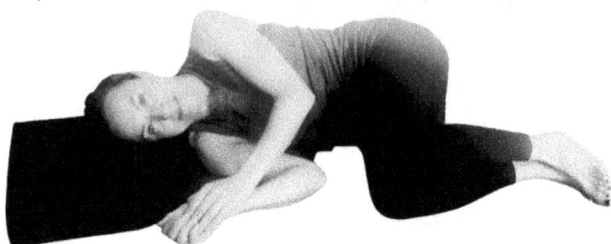

- Lie on your side and pull the hips and knees into a 90-degree angle.
- Place a pad under your head and a pad between the knees.
- Lips closed, gently place your tongue on the roof of the mouth.
- Breathe out and in through your nose.
- Exhale, inhale, and repeat for 1-2 minutes.
- Allow your breath to increase movement within your rib cage and back.

Head Control - Head Nods and Turns

Why?

- It's good to see where you are going!
- It activates your vestibular system.
- Moving the head reflexively turns on your core.
- It develops your self-awareness of any movement imbalances.

How?

Movement Position #1

FACE DOWN OR PRONE POSITION

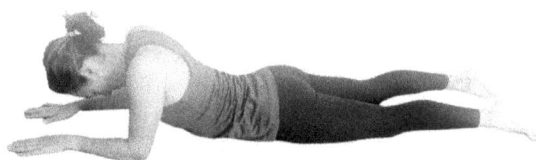

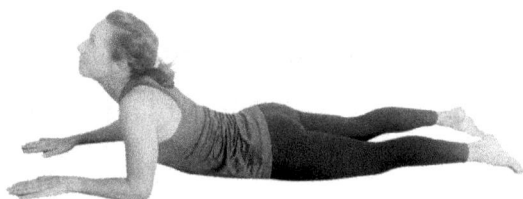

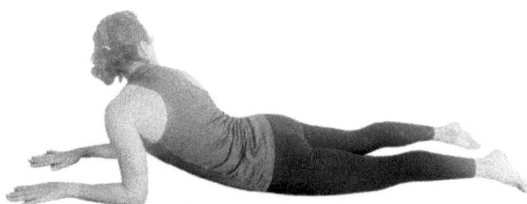

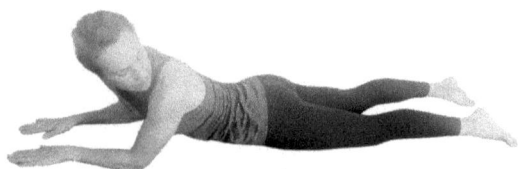

Pressing RESET for the Triathlete

Pay attention to how your body reflexively responds to the weight shift of your head. Notice how your back and abdominal muscles activate and respond.

Imagine you are looking for a sighting buoy in an open water swim. Restoring your original strength with head control can allow for better movement in the most stressful situations.

> **Restoring your original strength with head control can allow for better movement in the most stressful situations.**

- Lie face down.
- Lips closed, gently place your tongue on the roof of the mouth.
- Breathe out and in through your nose.
- Place yourself up onto your elbows.
- Lead with your eyes, look down, and nod your head down.
- Lead with your eyes, look up, and nod your head up.
- Lead with your eyes, look over your shoulder as you turn your head.
- Do it the other way.

Movement Position #2

SEATED QUADRUPED POSITION

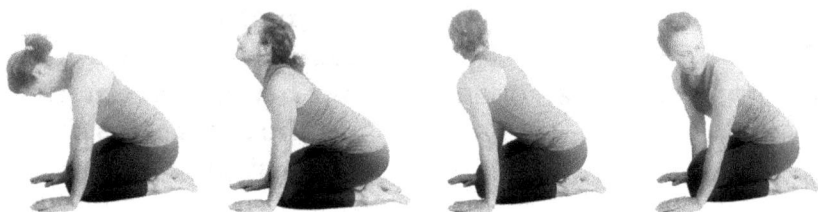

The seated quadruped position is specific to your sport. Being able to move your neck is important.

- Kneel on the floor on your hands and knees.

- Place a pad under the knees for comfort.

- Rock and sit back towards your feet. You can either point the toes straight backward or curl the toes forward.

- Lips closed, gently place your tongue on the roof of the mouth.

- Breathe out and in through your nose.

- Lead with your eyes, look down, and nod your head down.

- Lead with your eyes, look up, and nod your head up.

- Lead with your eyes, look over your shoulder as you turn your head.

- Do it the other way.

Movement Position #3

COMMANDO POSITION

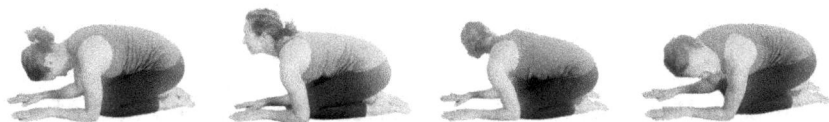

The commando position is specific to your sport. Being able to see where you are and what is around you is essential.

- Kneel on the floor on your hands and knees.
- Place a pad under the knees for comfort.
- Rock your hips back and lower them towards your feet. You can either point the toes straight backward or curl the toes forward.
- Lower yourself down onto your elbows.
- Lips closed, gently place your tongue on the roof of the mouth.
- Breathe out and in through your nose.
- Lead with your eyes, look down, and nod your head down.
- Lead with your eyes, look up, and nod your head up.
- Lead with your eyes, look over your shoulder as you turn your head.
- Do it the other way.

RESET #3

Rolling Patterns

Rolling patterns can feel great once you get the hang of them! They stretch you out and free you up.

Imagine how much better it is to wring out excess water from a towel by twisting it. Think of yourself as the towel. Roll away tension by gently rolling your body in different directions.

> **Roll away tension by gently rolling your body in different directions.**

Rolling patterns are achieved by contralateral signaling from your brain to your muscles. Even when some rolling patterns don't look like you are crossing your midline, you still use that reflexive wiring.

Rolling patterns turn on the core, priming the core to provide stability to the spine and pelvis reflexively. A stable spine can assist as you lengthen your stroke and glide through the water. It can anchor your seat to the bike as you push more power on the pedals.

The saying 'you can't shoot a cannon from a canoe' refers to the importance of having a strong core. If your core is strong, you can swim, bike, and run faster, as there are fewer energy leaks.

Why?

- It just feels good!

- It turns on your core.

- It's the foundation of contralateral movement.

- It frees up restrictions and positively influences your contralateral movement for all gait patterning.

- It restores movement to your rib cage and thoracic spine, improving shoulder mobility.

How?

Movement Position #1

ELBOW ROLLING

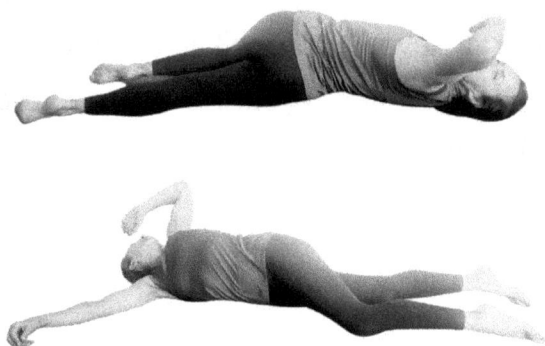

- Lie face down.
- Lips closed, gently place your tongue on the roof of the mouth.
- Breathe out and in through your nose.
- Reach the arms out in front of you on the floor.
- Lift your head and look over the right shoulder.
- Reach your right elbow up and back behind you.
- Allow the ribs to rotate.
- Relax your legs, leaving them in place.
- Repeat in the other direction.
- Breathe through any tension.
- Pay attention to any gains made in your movement.

Pressing RESET for the Triathlete

Movement Position #2

SEGMENTAL ROLLING - UPPER AND LOWER BODY

This rolling pattern builds off the elbow rolling. It fires the core and, again, just feels great!

You may find rolling leading with the legs feels easier. Focus on your breath when things get 'stuck'.

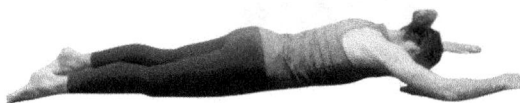

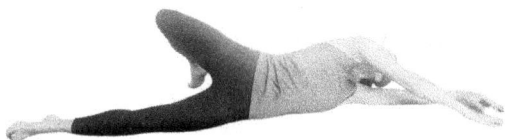

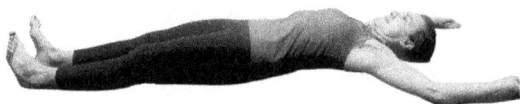

- Lie face down.
- Lips closed, gently place your tongue on the roof of the mouth.
- Breathe out and in through your nose.
- Relax the arms out in front of you on the floor.

- Lift your head and look back over your right shoulder.
- Reach your right arm or leg behind you, and allow yourself to roll over.
- Keep the rest of your body relaxed through the roll.
- Breathe through any tension.

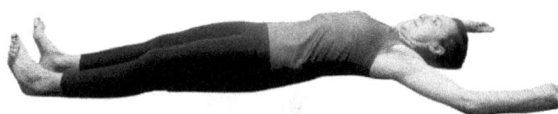

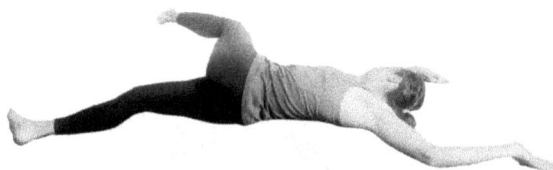

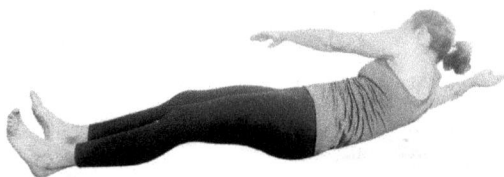

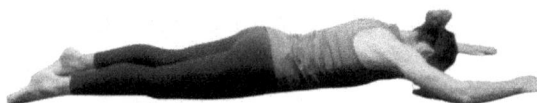

- Lie face up.
- Lips closed, gently place your tongue on the roof of the mouth.
- Breathe out and in through your nose.
- Relax the arms over your head on the floor.
- Lift your head, and look toward your right hip.
- Reach your right arm or leg across your body, and allow yourself to roll over.
- Keep the rest of your body relaxed through the roll.
- Breathe through any tension.

Movement Position #3

TORSO ROTATION

- Lie on your back, reach your arms out on the floor, perpendicular to your torso.

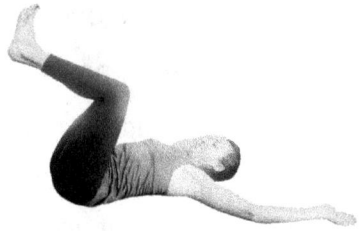

- Lips closed, gently place your tongue on the roof of the mouth.

- Breathe out and in through your nose.

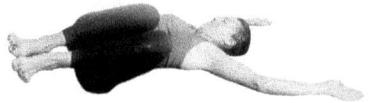

- Lift your feet, tuck your knees in over your belly button with your tailbone lifted.

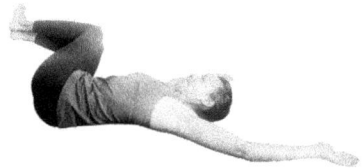

- Keeping shoulders flat on the floor, lower the knees to one side.

- Keep the knees together, pulled in close throughout the movement.

- Repeat to the other side as you exhale and inhale.

Pressing RESET for the Triathlete

Rocking Patterns

Why?

- It feels good.

- It turns on the core and ties the body together.

- It soothes the nervous system.

- Rocking promotes upper-body and lower-body mobility.

- It can be a gentle way to strengthen and mobilize the shoulders.

- It can become an effective strength movement with little to no equipment.

Movement Position #1

QUADRUPED ROCKING

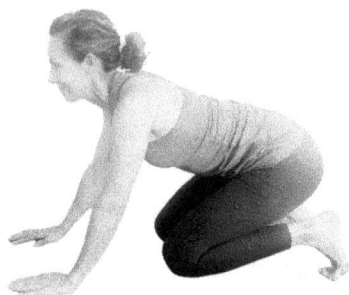

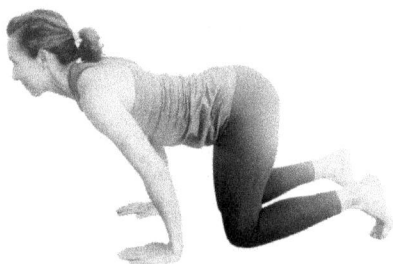

Rocking helps you find your tight spots. Play around with the placement of your knees and feet to help restore movement in those regions.

Rocking in different directions, such as forward and backward, in circles, and even in figures of eight, is not only good for the body but for your brain too.

How?

- On your hands and knees, look forward.
- Shoulders over hands, hips over knees, toes pointing backward or hooked under.
- Lips closed, gently place your tongue on the roof of the mouth.
- Breathe through your nose.
- Pressing your hands into the floor, rock your body backward.
- Pressing your hands into the floor, rock your body forward.
- Breathe through any tension.
- Keep the head up as you maintain a natural, neutral spine curvature.
- Explore rocking in different directions.

Movement Position #2

COMMANDO ROCKING

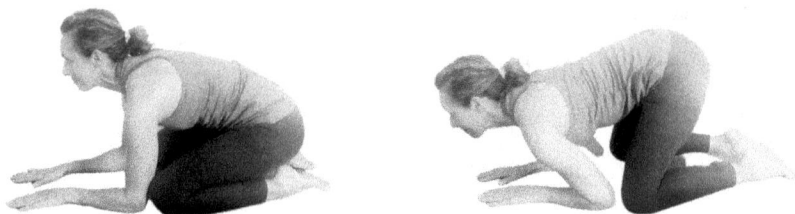

For a more sports specific position, try the commando rock. It may replicate the angles of your body position when in an aero position.

It fires up the core and turns on your shoulder stabilizers. It can be a gentle way to strengthen these areas, necessary for a swimmer's healthy shoulder.

• It can also become an effective strength movement when changed up a little and loading over time is added.

How?

• From a quadruped position, lower onto your elbows and look forward.

• Shoulders over elbows, hips over knees, toes pointing backward or hooked under.

Pressing RESET for the Triathlete

- Lips closed, gently place your tongue on the roof of the mouth.

- Breathe through your nose.

- Rock your body backward and forward.

- Breathe through any tension.

- Keep the head up as you maintain a natural, neutral spine curvature.

- Explore rocking in different directions.

Movement Position #3

SIDE LEG ROCKING

Although it seems there are no 'sideways' movement patterns in the sport of triathlon, it is important to maintain hip mobility. Gentle stretching with the leg out to the side can help with that.

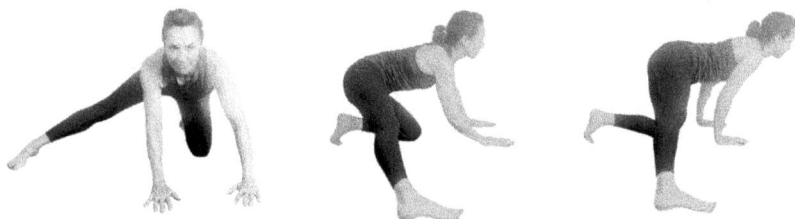

How?

- From a quadruped position, move one leg out to the side.
- Lips closed, gently place your tongue on the roof of the mouth.
- Breathe through your nose.
- Gently rock your body backward and forward.
- Breathe through any tension.
- Keep the head up as you maintain a natural, neutral spine curvature.

Movement Position #4

HEEL ROCKING

Having adequate ankle mobility is important for a great kick, a smooth pedal stroke, and a great tissue recoil during the foot strike and toe-off. As a triathlete, you need all of this!

> **Having adequate ankle mobility is important for a great kick**

Stretching the lower limb muscles and maintaining adequate ankle mobility is essential to help reduce your chances of injury.

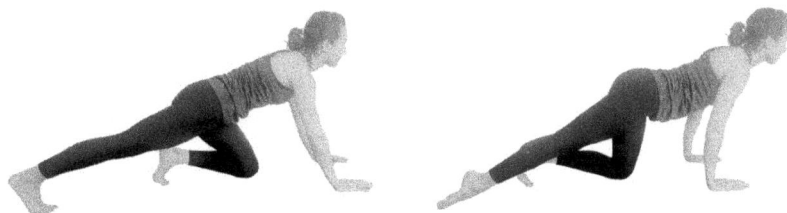

How?

- From a quadruped position, move one leg out straight behind you, toes hooked on the floor.
- Lips closed, gently place your tongue on the roof of the mouth.

- Breathe through your nose.
- Gently rock your body backward and forward.
- Breathe through any tension.
- Keep the head up as you maintain a natural, neutral spine curvature.

Contralateral Movements

Remember when I said you were wired to crawl from birth? But let's be real - how many of us actually carry on crawling as adolescents and adults of any age? If I told you why you should, would you?

Contralateral and crawling patterns not only provide super-strength gains but can build mental strength, too. 'Simply' crawling for a longer duration of time makes that clear quite quickly!

Crawling can go from a gentle form of strength training to a place where the whole body deals with unexpected and challenging forces. With consistent reinforcement of the gait pattern, your movement patterns can improve. Crawling could be your golden ticket to increasing your workload capacity as a multi-sporter. Trust me when I say it can produce incredible resilience and fortitude.

Why?

- It turns on connections throughout the whole body.
- It turns on the signaling of the brain.
- It can become an effective strength movement with little to no equipment.
- Smoother movement requires less effort.

Movement #1

BIRD DOG

Sports specific, the Bird Dog restores valuable movement and control to both the shoulder girdle and the hips. This gentle pattern restores strength, coordination, and timing, all beneficial to your swim, your posture on the bike, and your gait pattern.

Repeating this for a duration of 1-5 minutes brings phenomenal strength to the whole body.

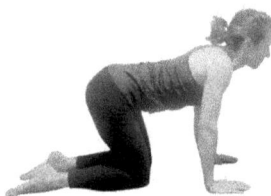

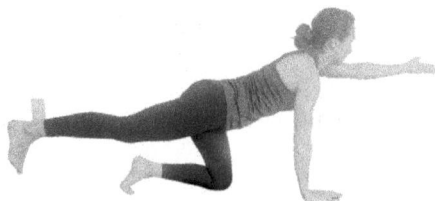

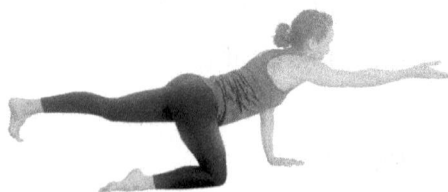

How?

- Get into a quadruped position; look forward.
- Lips closed, gently place your tongue on the roof of the mouth.
- Breathe through your nose.
- Move your left arm forward and right leg backward away from your body.
- Keep the head up as you maintain a natural, neutral curvature of the spine.
- Repeat with your right arm and left leg.
- Feel connected and move smoothly.

Movement #2

SKATER

Like the Bird Dog, except the arm sweeps back along your side. This movement helps reinforce the gait pattern. It can challenge the brain with a task in a different direction of coordination.

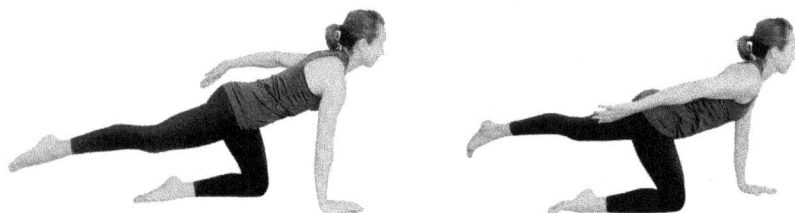

How?

- Get into a quadruped position; look forward.
- Lips closed, gently place your tongue on the roof of the mouth.
- Breathe through your nose.
- Move your left arm back along your side and your right leg backward behind you.
- Keep the head up as you maintain a natural, neutral spine curvature.
- Repeat with your right arm and left leg.
- Feel connected and move smoothly.

Movement #3

DYING BUG

This is another contralateral movement, lying on your back. Being on the back, this reflexively fires your abdominal muscles. Just by lifting your head slightly off the ground, you can perform an easy core workout.

While (hopefully) you won't be lying down on your back during your race, this contralateral pattern awakens your spine stabilizers as you also train the brain.

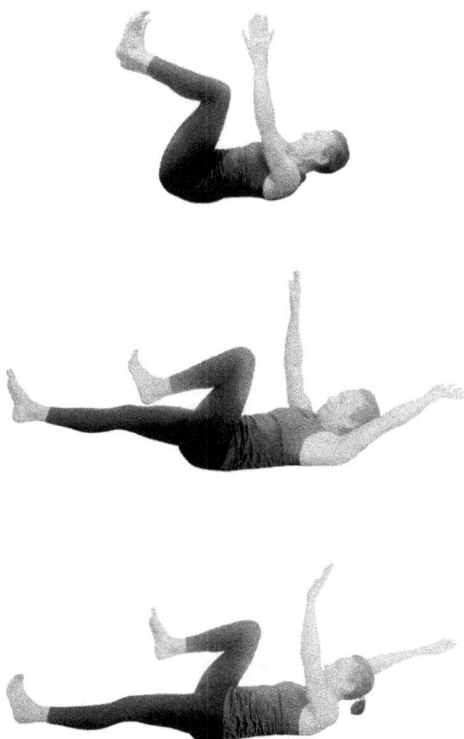

How?

- Lie on your back.
- Look towards your feet and lift your head slightly.
- Lips closed, gently place your tongue on the roof of the mouth.
- Breathe through your nose.
- Reach the arms up in the air above the shoulders.
- Bend your knees and bring your feet up off the floor.
- Keep the knees above your hips, tailbone slightly lifted.
- Lower your left arm behind your head and your right leg to the floor.
- Return that arm and leg to the air. Repeat with your other opposite limbs.
- Only move two limbs at a time.
- Always keep the knees over your hips.

Movement #4

HANDS AND KNEES CRAWLING

How?

- Get on your hands and knees; look forward.

- Lips closed, gently place your tongue on the roof of the mouth.

- Breathe through your nose.

- Pressing the hands into the floor, move your opposite arms and legs together to crawl forward or backward.

- Keep the head up as you maintain a natural, neutral spine curvature.

- Stop and RESET the diaphragm nasal breathing as soon as you lose the contralateral pattern.

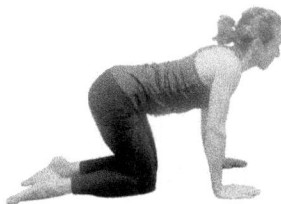

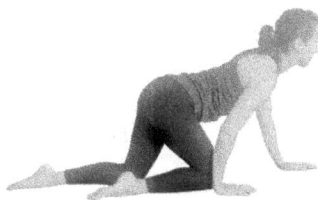

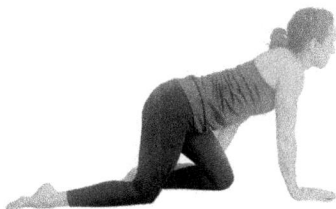

Movement #5

LEOPARD CRAWLING

This is a progression from the hands and knees crawl.

How?

- From your hands and knees position, lift the knees slightly off the floor; look forward.

- Lips closed, gently place your tongue on the roof of the mouth.

- Breathe through your nose.

- Pressing the hands into the floor, move your opposite arms and legs together to crawl forward or backward.

- Keep your hips low and chest open.

- Keep the head up as you maintain a natural, neutral spine curvature.

- Stop and RESET the diaphragm nasal breathing as soon as you lose the contralateral pattern.

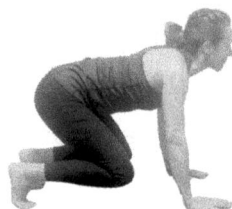

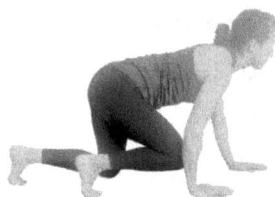

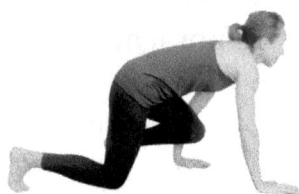

Movement #6

CROSS CRAWLS

Cross crawls are a convenient way to turn on the brain without lying down!

Done seated, kneeling, standing, or marching, you can use these as an effective way to wake up your brain.

> **Discover fun ways to add directional changes**

As a warm-up, cool-down, or used as part of a recovery between hard run intervals, they can reset your gait pattern. Discover fun ways to add directional changes, such as moving forward, backward, sideways, and in circles.

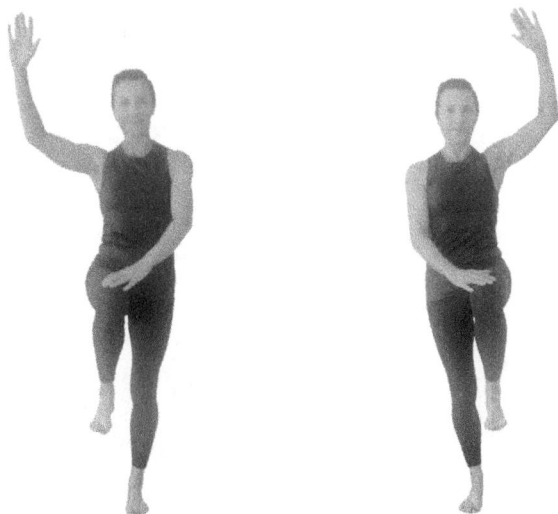

How?

- Try first from a seated position, then a tall kneeling position, and finally a standing position.
- Lips closed, gently place your tongue on the roof of the mouth.
- Breathe through your nose.
- Keep a tall spine looking forward.
- Touch your opposite limbs together.
- Keep your toes up when possible.
- Progress to moving in different directions.

Putting It All Together

As long as you include the Three Pillars (diaphragmatic breathing, moving your head, and moving contralaterally), there is no wrong order. There is no fixed algorithm for the sequence of the RESETs.

In the world of Original Strength, we like to say, "Meet yourself where you are at," - meaning go with the

> **Meet yourself where you are at.**

RESETs that feel good for you at that time. You will become your own expert with what works for you.

Some of you will find more benefit from rocking than rolling at times and visa versa. One rolling pattern may work better that day than another. You will feel different daily, just as you do in your training sessions.

Use RESETs for any and all of the following:

- Warm up before a training session.
- Cool down after a training session.
- Strength routine.
- Restoration between training sessions and recovery days.
- Daily feel-good practice.

Suggested Pre-Swim RESET Routine

Perform each movement for 1-2 minutes.

- Face down diaphragmatic nasal breathing
- Prone position head nods and turns
- Segmental upper and lower body rolling
- Quadruped rocking
- Heel rocking
- Bird dog with head nods and turns at any time
- Dying bug
- Standing cross crawls

Suggested Pre-Bike RESET Routine

Perform each movement for 1-2 minutes.

- Diaphragmatic nasal breathing in a seated quadruped position
- Head nods and turns in a seated quadruped position
- Elbow rolling
- Torso rotation
- Commando rocking, add more head nods and turns
- Side leg rocking

- Bird dog
- Hands and knees crawling

Suggested Pre-Run RESET Routine

Perform each movement for 1-2 minutes.

- Side lying 90-90 diaphragmatic nasal breathing, adding in head nods and turns
- Upper and lower body rolling patterns
- Quadruped rocking in all directions
- Heel rocking
- Skater
- Standing to marching cross crawl

If you want to use the same routine as a cool down, simply reverse the order, finishing with the breathing.

Sample Training Session

It is possible to build strength using RESETs. There are many ways to increase their challenge. Increasing the load through a change of body position or adding resistance or a load can lead to a rewarding workout.

Below is just one routine shown; if done just 2 or 3 days a week, it can be an effective way to gain strength. It does not require much time and does not need expensive equipment.

General Guidelines

- Perform each movement for 1 minute.
- Repeat the whole routine for a total of 3 rounds.
- Maintain nasal breathing as much as possible.
- Choose any gentle RESET to recover for 1 minute between rounds to restore nasal breathing.

Sample Routine

- Diaphragmatic breathing with head nods and turns from a quadruped position
- Rolling to standing

  Progression: After completing a roll of your choice, stand up in a different pattern each time, get back down on the floor and repeat.

Recovery with 20 super slow Standing Cross Crawls

- Hands and knees rocking to elevated rocking

  Progression: With your knees slightly off the floor, slowly rock your hips back and forward to a plank position; look forwards.

- Torso rotation

  Progression: With the knees above your belly button and legs together, slowly move side to side. Hold off the ground in the lowest position. Keep shoulder blades down on the floor.

Recovery with 20 super slow Standing cross crawls

- Dying bug

  Progression: Head up, tailbone up, hold a ball in both hands and reach back in opposition to the moving leg.

- Leopard crawling

  Progression: Super slow crawl, hover, and move over the ground. Try moving in different directions as you keep your head up, looking forward.

And Finally,

Over the past two decades, I have Pressed RESET within my daily practice, both as a health and fitness professional and as a competitive endurance athlete.

They have helped me grow my business training platform and helped me fully recover from two major surgeries.

I have seen the restoration of movement within my clients, and I have experienced it personally.

Try them by adding them to your daily practice. Daily practice can bring about discoveries.

> **Use RESETs to calm race day nerves**

Use RESETs to calm race day nerves, improve postural durability, and help build a run gait that feels smoother and more 'tied' together.

Become your own keeper of the RESETs; your body and nervous system will thank you for it.

Allow them to add balance to your work and play. By doing so, I hope you experience performance breakthroughs for that important day.

No matter what you are racing for, the podium or to finish your first triathlon, I wish you much success and fortitude.

About Our Contributor:

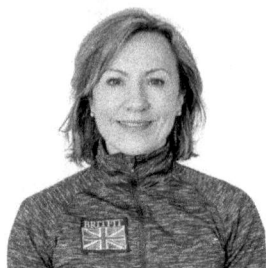

Jackie Miller, owner of Britfit Personal Training & Coaching, has worked in the Health and Fitness Industry for over 25 years.

Through those years, she has worked with many clients, from recreational to high-performance athletes.

Her credentials represent her understanding of sports science and movement. Applying that knowledge results in delivering a training system specifically designed for her clients' needs.

CREDENTIALS

- USA Triathlon Level III Coach
- FMS Level 1 and 2 certified
- Original Strength Certified PRO
- ACE Personal Trainer

SERVICES OFFERED

- Personalized Training Programming: Fitness plans to high-performance endurance sports training plans for seasonal coaching

- Personal Training: In-person and virtual
- Customized Wellness Programs
- Public Speaking
- Available nationally and internationally

BACKGROUND

Jackie Miller is proud to be a female small business owner.

Britfit has grown to meet the industry's diversifying direction since Jackie's early years as a personal trainer at the YMCA in Charlotte, North Carolina.

Her business has expanded into a strong team of clients, including many high-performance athletes and recreational fitness clients of all ages and abilities.

Jackie still loves to compete as an All-American Ranked Triathlete and Duathlete in long-distance events.

As a Team USA athlete, she has brought home a gold and two silver medals from ITU- World Triathlon Championship events.

Her passion for endurance racing credits her with several top 3 140.6 distance IronMan podium wins and several 70.3 distance IronMan World Championship finishes.

Want to learn more?

This booklet was designed to give a brief overview of the Original Strength System and how it can help you Press RESET to become an even better triathlete.

We put it together because we know it can help everyone and anyone. If you do nothing more than what is in this booklet, you will notice many changes in how your mind and body begin to feel and react to various situations.

Original Strength is a nervous system restoration company with a mission to bring hope and strength of movement to every body in the world. It provides quality continuing education courses and books to health & fitness and education professionals to enhance their knowledge and provide their patients, clients, athletes, and students with better outcomes. Based on the human developmental sequence and the human body's design, the Original Strength System teaches movements that help RESET an individual's neuromuscular system, allowing them to enjoy improved physical movement and physiological function.

If you want to know more about Pressing RESET and regaining your original strength, visit https://originalstrength.net. There, you will find various books, hundreds of free video tutorials (**OS Movement Snax**), and a complete listing of our courses and OS Certified Professionals near you.

If you're looking to improve your movement system, consider seeking out an OS Certified Professional. They can perform an Original Strength Screen and Assessment (OSSA), which is a fast and simple method for identifying areas to unlock your potential. With the OSSA, the professional can determine the most effective starting point for your journey towards restoring your Original Strength through the Pressing RESET technique.

We encourage you to contact the OS team with any questions you may have. ***Please keep us updated with your progress; we really want to know how you are doing - progress@OriginalStrength.net.***

Press RESET now and live life better & stronger because you were awesomely and wonderfully made to accomplish amazing things.

For more information:

⏻riginal
strength

Original Strength Systems, LLC
OriginalStrength.net

PressingRESETfor@Originalstrength.net